HOW TO GUIDE: CLOBETASOL PROPIONATE

A definitive Handbook on how to reduce swelling, redness, itching, or rashes caused by skin conditions, such as eczema and psoriasis

Dr. Philips Judy

Table of Contents

INTRODUCTION 3

    OVERVIEW OF CLOBETASOL PROPIONATE 3

    Definition and Chemical Structure...3

    History and Development...4

    Purpose of the Book 4

CHAPTER 1: UNDERSTANDING CLOBETASOL PROPIONATE.................................6

    MECHANISM OF ACTION 6

    Pharmacokinetics and Pharmacodynamics 7

    Forms and Formulations 8

CHAPTER 2: MEDICAL USES AND INDICATIONS 11

    SKIN CONDITIONS TREATED BY CLOBETASOL PROPIONATE.......................11

    Eczema 11

    Dermatitis 12

    Lichen Planus 13

    Other Indications 13

    Off-Label Uses...14

    Comparative Effectiveness 14

    Summary..15

CHAPTER 3: APPLICATION AND ADMINISTRATION..17

    PROPER USAGE GUIDELINES..17

    Application Techniques 17

    Frequency and Duration of Use 19

    Pediatric Use...20

    Use in Pregnancy and Lactation...20

    Elderly Patients 21

    Summary..21

CHAPTER 4: SAFETY AND SIDE EFFECTS 23

COMMON SIDE EFFECTS 23

Dryness and Cracking..23

Thinning of the Skin 24

Serious Adverse Reactions 24

Hypothalamic-Pituitary-Adrenal (HPA) Axis Suppression 24

Cushing's Syndrome 25

Allergic Reactions 26

Managing Side Effects...26

When to Seek Medical Attention 27

Summary...28

CONCLUSION 29

OVERVIEW OF CLOBETASOL PROPIONATE

Clobetasol propionate is a potent topical corticosteroid used primarily to treat various skin conditions. It is renowned for its anti-inflammatory and immunosuppressive properties, which make it highly effective in reducing symptoms such as itching, redness, and swelling. This introduction aims to provide a foundational understanding of clobetasol propionate, setting the stage for a comprehensive exploration of its uses, benefits, and potential risks.

Definition and Chemical Structure

Clobetasol propionate is a synthetic corticosteroid belonging to the class of medications known as glucocorticoids. It is chemically described as 21-chloro-9-fluoro-11β,17-dihydroxy-16β-methylpregna-1,4-diene-3,20-dione 17-propionate. Its molecular formula is $C_{25}H_{32}ClFO_5$, and it has a molecular weight of 466.97 g/mol. The structure of clobetasol propionate includes a corticosteroid nucleus with a chlorine and fluorine substitution, enhancing its potency compared to other corticosteroids.

History and Development

Clobetasol propionate was first synthesized in the late 20th century as part of the ongoing efforts to develop more effective and potent corticosteroids for dermatological use. Its introduction marked a significant advancement in the treatment of severe inflammatory skin conditions. The development process involved rigorous clinical testing to establish its efficacy and safety profile, leading to its approval by various health authorities worldwide.

Purpose of the Book

This book is designed to serve as an authoritative resource on clobetasol propionate, providing detailed information on its pharmacology, clinical applications, and safety considerations. It aims to educate healthcare professionals, patients, and researchers on the appropriate use of this medication, helping to optimize treatment outcomes and minimize adverse effects. By offering a thorough understanding of clobetasol propionate, this book seeks to enhance patient care and support informed decision-making in clinical practice.

Through this introduction, readers will gain a preliminary insight into the significance of clobetasol propionate in dermatology, paving the way for a deeper dive into its various aspects in the subsequent chapters. Whether you are a medical professional looking to expand your knowledge or a patient seeking to understand your treatment options, this book will provide you with valuable information and practical guidance.

MECHANISM OF ACTION

Clobetasol propionate is a potent glucocorticoid, which exerts its therapeutic effects through several mechanisms. It primarily works by binding to glucocorticoid receptors in the cytoplasm of target cells. This binding initiates a cascade of events leading to the translocation of the receptor-ligand complex into the cell nucleus, where it interacts with specific DNA sequences to regulate the transcription of glucocorticoid-responsive genes. These genes encode proteins that mediate anti-inflammatory and immunosuppressive effects, such as lipocortins, which inhibit phospholipase A2, reducing the synthesis of pro-inflammatory mediators like prostaglandins and leukotrienes. Additionally, clobetasol propionate decreases the production of cytokines and other inflammatory markers, thereby reducing inflammation and immune responses.

Pharmacokinetics and Pharmacodynamics

Pharmacokinetics describes how the drug is absorbed, distributed, metabolized, and excreted in the body. Clobetasol propionate, when applied topically, is absorbed through the skin. Its absorption rate depends on various factors, including the integrity of the skin barrier, the presence of inflammation or disease, and the formulation of the product. Once absorbed, clobetasol propionate undergoes extensive metabolism primarily in the liver, and its metabolites are excreted in the urine.

Pharmacodynamics involves the effects of the drug on the body. Clobetasol propionate's high potency is due to its strong binding affinity to glucocorticoid receptors, resulting in pronounced anti-inflammatory effects even at low concentrations. Its effectiveness in reducing symptoms of inflammation and immune responses makes it a valuable treatment option for severe dermatological conditions.

Forms and Formulations

Topical Creams and Ointments

Topical creams and ointments are the most common formulations of clobetasol propionate. Creams are generally preferred for moist or weeping lesions due to their hydrophilic nature, while ointments are more suitable for dry, scaly lesions because of their occlusive properties, which help retain moisture in the skin.

Lotions, Gels, and Sprays

Lotions and gels provide an alternative for patients who prefer a lighter, non-greasy formulation. These are particularly useful for hairy areas of the body, such as the scalp, where creams and ointments may be difficult to apply. Sprays offer an additional advantage of easy application over large or hard-to-reach areas.

Shampoos and Foams

Shampoos and foams are specifically formulated for scalp conditions. They provide a convenient option for treating conditions like scalp psoriasis or seborrheic dermatitis, ensuring even distribution and better patient compliance.

In summary, clobetasol propionate is available in various formulations to cater to different types of skin conditions and patient preferences, enhancing its versatility and effectiveness as a treatment option.

Chapter 1 provides a foundational understanding of clobetasol propionate, detailing its mechanism of action, pharmacokinetics, pharmacodynamics, and the various forms in which it is available. This comprehensive overview sets the stage for the subsequent chapters, which will delve deeper into the clinical applications, safety considerations, and practical aspects of using clobetasol propionate. By understanding the basics, readers can better appreciate the complexities and nuances of this powerful medication, leading to more informed and effective use.

SKIN CONDITIONS TREATED BY CLOBETASOL PROPIONATE

Psoriasis is a chronic autoimmune condition characterized by the rapid turnover of skin cells, leading to the formation of thick, red, scaly patches. Clobetasol propionate is often prescribed for moderate to severe plaque psoriasis due to its potent anti-inflammatory and immunosuppressive properties. It helps to reduce the redness, scaling, and thickness of psoriatic plaques, providing relief from the associated itching and discomfort. Treatment with clobetasol propionate can significantly improve the quality of life for psoriasis patients by controlling flare-ups and maintaining remission.

Eczema

Eczema, or atopic dermatitis, is a condition marked by inflamed, itchy, and cracked skin. Clobetasol propionate is typically reserved for short-term use in severe cases of eczema or for managing acute flare-ups. Its potent anti-inflammatory effects help to rapidly reduce symptoms, allowing the skin to heal and preventing secondary infections that can result from scratching and broken skin barriers. However, due to its strength, it is often used as part of a broader eczema management plan that includes milder corticosteroids and non-steroidal treatments for long-term control.

Dermatitis

Various forms of dermatitis, such as contact dermatitis and seborrheic dermatitis, can also be effectively treated with clobetasol propionate. In contact dermatitis, which is caused by exposure to allergens or irritants, clobetasol propionate reduces the inflammatory response, alleviating symptoms like redness, swelling, and itching. In seborrheic dermatitis, it helps control the inflammatory components and reduces the severity of symptoms, especially in resistant cases where other treatments have failed.

Lichen Planus

Lichen planus is a relatively rare skin condition characterized by purplish, itchy, flat-topped bumps, often appearing on the wrists, lower back, and ankles. Clobetasol propionate is effective in managing lichen planus by reducing inflammation and suppressing the immune response that contributes to the formation of these lesions. Regular application can help to clear the lesions and relieve the itching and discomfort associated with this condition.

Other Indications

Clobetasol propionate is also used to treat a variety of other dermatological conditions, including discoid lupus erythematosus, granuloma annulare, and vitiligo. In each of these conditions, the medication's potent anti-inflammatory and immunosuppressive properties help to manage symptoms and prevent disease progression.

Off-Label Uses

Beyond its approved indications, clobetasol propionate is sometimes used off-label for other inflammatory and autoimmune conditions. For instance, it has been investigated for use in treating alopecia areata, a condition characterized by sudden hair loss due to an autoimmune attack on hair follicles. While not formally approved for this indication, some studies suggest that clobetasol propionate can help to stimulate hair regrowth in affected areas by reducing local inflammation and immune activity.

Comparative Effectiveness

Comparing the effectiveness of clobetasol propionate with other treatments is essential for optimizing patient care. Studies have shown that clobetasol propionate is generally more effective than lower-potency corticosteroids in rapidly controlling severe inflammatory skin conditions. However, its high potency also increases the risk of side effects, making it crucial to balance effectiveness with safety. In some cases, combining clobetasol propionate with other therapies, such as systemic immunosuppressants or biologics, can provide enhanced results while minimizing adverse effects.

Summary

Chapter 2 highlights the wide range of skin conditions that can be effectively treated with clobetasol propionate, emphasizing its versatility and potency as a therapeutic agent. From common conditions like psoriasis and eczema to more specialized uses in lichen planus and off-label applications, clobetasol propionate plays a crucial role in dermatological care. The chapter also underscores the importance of comparative effectiveness studies in guiding clinical decisions and optimizing treatment outcomes for patients with severe or refractory skin conditions.

CHAPTER 3: APPLICATION AND ADMINISTRATION

PROPER USAGE GUIDELINES

The correct dosage of clobetasol propionate is crucial for achieving the desired therapeutic effect while minimizing the risk of side effects. Typically, clobetasol propionate should be applied in a thin layer to the affected area(s) of the skin once or twice daily. The specific frequency and duration of application depend on the severity of the condition and the response to treatment. It is important to follow the prescribing physician's instructions carefully. Overuse or prolonged use can lead to adverse effects, including skin thinning and systemic absorption leading to more serious side effects.

Application Techniques

Proper application techniques ensure maximum efficacy and minimize potential side effects:

1. **Clean and Dry the Affected Area**: Before applying clobetasol propionate, clean and dry the affected area thoroughly. This removes any dirt or debris that might interfere with the medication's absorption.

2. **Apply a Thin Layer**: Use a small amount of clobetasol propionate and spread it in a thin, even layer over the affected area. Gently rub it into the skin until it is fully absorbed.

3. **Wash Hands**: After application, wash your hands thoroughly to prevent the medication from spreading to other areas of your body or to other individuals.

4. **Avoid Occlusion**: Unless specifically directed by a healthcare provider, avoid covering the treated area with bandages, dressings, or tight clothing, as

occlusion can increase the risk of systemic absorption and side effects.

5. **Follow Specific Instructions for Different Formulations**: Different formulations (creams, ointments, lotions, gels, sprays, shampoos, and foams) may have specific application instructions. For example, foams and sprays should be shaken well before use, and shampoos should be left on the scalp for a prescribed duration before rinsing.

Frequency and Duration of Use

Clobetasol propionate is typically used for short-term treatment due to its high potency. The duration of treatment should generally not exceed two to four weeks without medical supervision. For chronic conditions, intermittent use or cycling with lower-potency corticosteroids may be recommended to reduce the risk of side effects. Continuous long-term use is discouraged to avoid potential complications like skin atrophy and HPA axis suppression.

Pediatric Use

Clobetasol propionate is not generally recommended for use in children due to the increased risk of systemic absorption and side effects. However, in certain severe cases, it may be prescribed with caution. When used in pediatric patients, it is crucial to use the lowest effective dose for the shortest duration possible, and regular monitoring by a healthcare provider is essential.

Use in Pregnancy and Lactation

The safety of clobetasol propionate during pregnancy and lactation has not been fully established. It should only be used during pregnancy if the potential benefits justify the potential risks to the fetus. During lactation, it is advisable to avoid applying clobetasol propionate to the breast area to prevent accidental ingestion by the nursing infant.

Consultation with a healthcare provider is recommended to weigh the risks and benefits in these situations.

Elderly Patients

Elderly patients may have increased susceptibility to the adverse effects of topical corticosteroids due to thinner skin and potential for comorbid conditions. Lower potency corticosteroids or less frequent application may be considered for elderly patients, and regular monitoring for side effects is advised.

Summary

Chapter 3 provides comprehensive guidelines on the proper application and administration of clobetasol propionate. By understanding the correct dosage, application techniques, and special considerations for different patient populations, healthcare providers and patients can maximize the therapeutic benefits of clobetasol propionate while minimizing potential risks. The chapter emphasizes the importance of adhering to prescribed instructions and regularly consulting with healthcare providers to ensure safe and effective treatment.

COMMON SIDE EFFECTS

One of the most frequently reported side effects of clobetasol propionate is skin irritation at the site of application. This can manifest as redness, itching, burning, or stinging. Such reactions are usually mild and transient, resolving after a short period of continued use. However, if irritation persists or worsens, discontinuation and consultation with a healthcare provider are advisable.

Dryness and Cracking

Clobetasol propionate can cause the skin to become excessively dry, leading to peeling, flaking, and cracking. This side effect is particularly common with prolonged use. Moisturizers or emollients may help alleviate dryness and protect the skin barrier. Patients should be advised to apply these products after the medication has been absorbed.

Thinning of the Skin

Long-term use of clobetasol propionate can result in skin atrophy or thinning. This side effect occurs because corticosteroids can inhibit collagen synthesis, weakening the structural integrity of the skin. Thinned skin is more prone to bruising, tearing, and the development of stretch marks (striae). To minimize this risk, clobetasol propionate should be used for the shortest duration necessary to achieve the desired therapeutic effect.

Serious Adverse Reactions

Hypothalamic-Pituitary-Adrenal (HPA) Axis Suppression

Clobetasol propionate, especially when used over large surface areas or under occlusive dressings, can be absorbed systemically and potentially suppress the HPA axis. This suppression can lead to decreased production of endogenous corticosteroids, resulting in symptoms like fatigue, hypotension, and adrenal crisis in severe cases. To monitor for HPA axis suppression, healthcare providers may conduct periodic tests, such as measuring morning serum cortisol levels. Gradual tapering of the medication rather than abrupt discontinuation can help mitigate the risk of adrenal insufficiency.

Cushing's Syndrome

Cushing's syndrome is a rare but serious side effect of prolonged high-dose corticosteroid therapy, including clobetasol propionate. Symptoms include weight gain, fatty deposits around the face and neck (moon face), thinning skin, muscle weakness, and elevated blood sugar levels. If signs of Cushing's syndrome develop, the use of clobetasol propionate should be reevaluated, and alternative treatments should be considered.

Allergic Reactions

Although uncommon, some patients may experience allergic reactions to clobetasol propionate. These reactions can range from mild contact dermatitis to severe anaphylactic responses. Symptoms include rash, itching, swelling, dizziness, and difficulty breathing. Immediate medical attention is required if an allergic reaction occurs, and the medication should be discontinued.

Managing Side Effects

Effective management of side effects involves regular monitoring and preventive measures:

1. **Regular Follow-Ups**: Patients using clobetasol propionate, especially for extended periods, should have regular follow-up appointments with their healthcare provider to monitor for side effects and assess treatment efficacy.

2. **Skin Care**: Maintaining good skin care practices, such as using gentle cleansers and moisturizers, can help prevent and manage dryness and irritation.

3. **Avoiding Occlusive Dressings**: Unless specifically instructed by a healthcare provider, patients should avoid using occlusive dressings, which can increase the risk of systemic absorption and side effects.

4. **Educating Patients**: Patients should be educated about the potential side effects of clobetasol propionate and instructed to report any unusual symptoms promptly.

When to Seek Medical Attention

Patients should be advised to seek medical attention if they experience:

- Severe or persistent skin irritation

- Symptoms of HPA axis suppression, such as fatigue or weakness

- Signs of Cushing's syndrome, such as weight gain or unusual fat distribution

- Any signs of an allergic reaction, including rash, swelling, or difficulty breathing

Summary

Chapter 4 emphasizes the importance of understanding and managing the potential side effects of clobetasol propionate to ensure safe and effective use. By being aware of common and serious adverse reactions, patients and healthcare providers can take proactive steps to monitor and mitigate these risks. Regular follow-ups, patient education, and adherence to prescribed usage guidelines are key strategies for minimizing side effects and maximizing the therapeutic benefits of clobetasol propionate.

CONCLUSION

Clobetasol propionate is a highly potent corticosteroid that plays a crucial role in the management of various inflammatory and autoimmune skin conditions. Its efficacy in reducing symptoms such as redness, swelling, and itching makes it a valuable tool for dermatologists and patients alike. However, with its high potency comes the need for careful use and vigilant monitoring to avoid potential adverse effects.

Throughout this book, we have explored the comprehensive aspects of clobetasol propionate, from its pharmacological mechanisms and various formulations to its medical uses, safety considerations, and proper administration techniques. Understanding these facets helps ensure that clobetasol propionate is used effectively and safely, providing relief to patients while minimizing the risk of side effects.

Key points to remember include:

1. **Versatile Applications**: Clobetasol propionate is effective in treating a wide range of skin conditions, including psoriasis, eczema, dermatitis, and lichen planus. Its versatility extends to off-label uses and investigational treatments, showcasing its broad therapeutic potential.

2. **Proper Application and Administration**: Following dosage instructions and proper application techniques is essential to maximize the medication's benefits while reducing the risk of side effects. Special considerations are necessary for different patient populations, including children, pregnant or lactating women, and the elderly.

3. **Safety and Side Effects**: Awareness and management of potential side effects, ranging from common skin irritation to serious systemic effects like HPA axis

suppression and Cushing's syndrome, are critical. Regular monitoring and patient education are key strategies in ensuring safe use.

4. **Comparative Effectiveness**: Clobetasol propionate's high potency requires careful comparison with other treatments to balance efficacy and safety. Combining it with other therapies may enhance results while minimizing adverse effects.

Looking ahead, ongoing research and development continue to refine our understanding of clobetasol propionate, leading to innovations in formulation and new therapeutic applications. As we advance, the insights gained from clinical practice and research will further optimize the use of this powerful medication, improving patient outcomes and enhancing the quality of life for those affected by severe dermatological conditions.

In conclusion, clobetasol propionate remains an indispensable component of dermatological therapy. By adhering to best practices in its application and administration, healthcare providers can harness its full potential while safeguarding patient health. This book aims to serve as a comprehensive resource, equipping readers with the knowledge needed to effectively and safely utilize clobetasol propionate in clinical practice.

THE END

www.ingramcontent.com/pod-product-compliance
Lightning Source LLC
Chambersburg PA
CBHW081812250726
48653CB00010B/3915